Motivational Interviewing Training for Health Professionals

Christine W. Thorpe EdD, EdM,CHES

Contents

Introduction

Definition of Motivational Interviewing

Motivational Interviewing Theory

General Principles of MI

  1. Express Empathy
  2. Support Self-Efficacy
  3. Roll with Resistance
  4. Develop Discrepancy
  5. Avoid Argumentation

Stages of Learning Motivational Interviewing

  1. openness to collaboration with patients' own expertise
  2. proficiency in patient-centered counseling, including accurate empathy
  3. recognition of key aspects of patient speech that guide the practice of MI
  4. eliciting and strengthening patient change talk
  5. rolling with resistance
  6. negotiating change plans
  7. consolidating patient commitment
  8. switching flexibly between MI and other intervention styles

Motivational Interviewing Strategies and Statements

Appendix

Case Studies

9 Tips for Motivational Interviewing Success

Addressing Motivational Interviewing Resistance from Staff

Bibliography

Introduction

Motivation, a reason or drive toward a particular act, is a dynamic and purposeful step on behalf of the patient. This step is taken in partnership with the health professional who guides the patient toward intentional change. The utilization of motivational interviewing among health care providers has continued to increase since its development in 1983 by Professors William Miller and Stephen Rollnick. Motivational interviewing has shown success in addressing addictions; prenatal smoking cessation; alcohol substance abuse; eating disorders; and risky sexual behavior. The spirit of Motivational Interviewing appreciates the opportunity for behavior change in collaboration with the patient.

The purpose of this workbook is to train health professionals in advancing their knowledge and skills in guiding behavior change among your patients. Your openness to this conversational style will enable you to truly utilize the skills you will be presented today.

During this training, participants will have the opportunity to:

- Demonstrate understanding of change theory and motivational strategies
- Become familiar with the principles and components of motivational interviewing
- Learning guidelines for applying motivational interviewing techniques
- Demonstrate basic skills for enhancing client motivation

Through presentations, discussions, interactives exercises and role-playing, each participant will have an opportunity to learn approaches to motivational interviewing. At the end of this workbook you will find resources to support you in the workplace, as well as a list of publications about motivational interviewing.

Motivational Interviewing

Definition:

According to researchers William Miller and Stephen Rollnick (1991), "*motivational interviewing is a directive, client-centered counseling style for eliciting behavior change by helping clients to explore and resolve ambivalence*" (p. 325).

Motivational Interviewing: What it is and what it is not

MI is:	MI is not:
a conversation about change	the stages of change model
utilized to evoke personal motivation for change	a way of tricking people into doing what you want them to do
collaborative	a technique
used to help people make their own decisions	a decision based on a simple list of pros and cons
purposeful	assessment feedback
goal-oriented	cognitive-behavior therapy (psychotherapy)
(uses) specific helping skills	client-centered therapy (talk therapy)
guided by specific aspects of patient language	easy to learn
(supports) elaboration, affirmation, reflection and summary of patient language	practice as usual
not resistant to patient resistance	a remedy for all difficulties

MI Theory

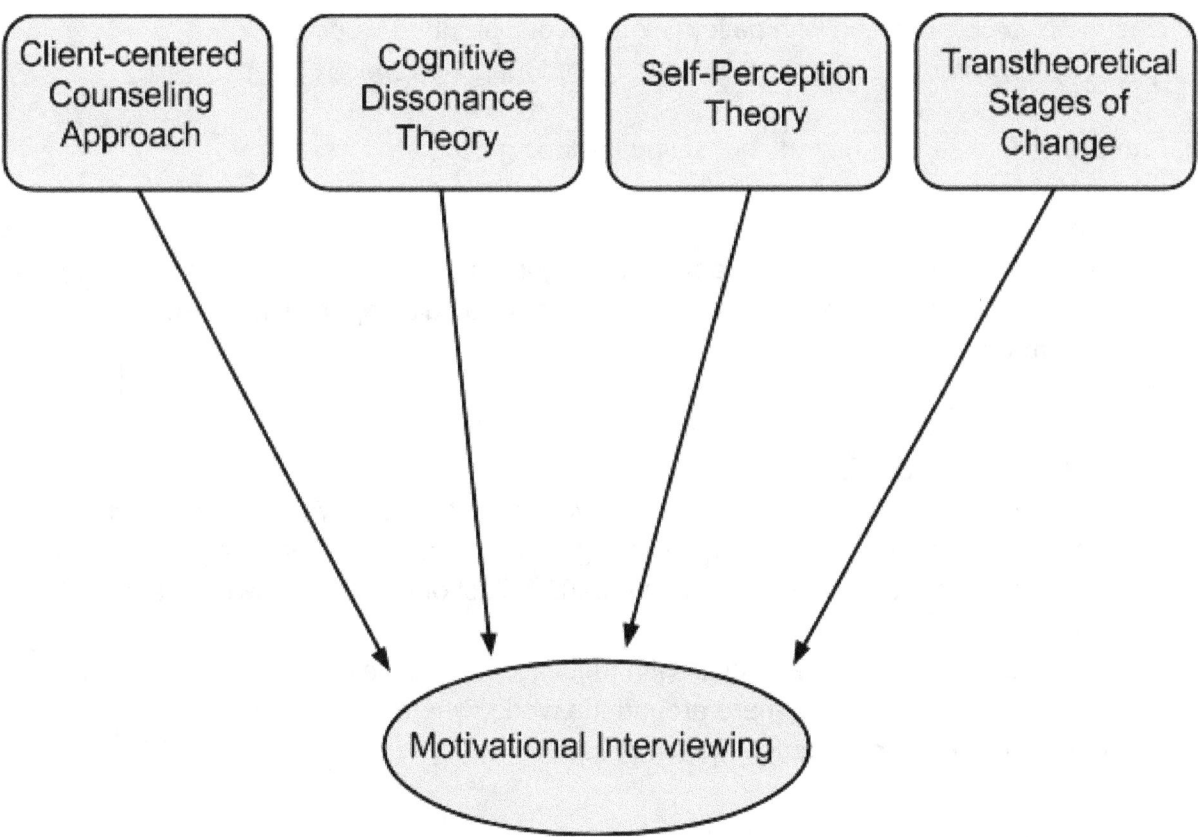

The General Principles of MI:

1. Express Empathy - influences patient behavior change.

2. Support Self-Efficacy - what is this the patient's
   Desire
   Ability
   Reasons
   Need
   Commitment
to change, and what is their strength for each of these areas by the end of the session.

3. Roll with Resistance - supports gentle guidance of the patient.

4. Develop Discrepancy - reflectively listening to patient's perspective.

5. Avoid Argumentation - affirm the feelings of the patient.

Stages of Learning MI

1. Openness to collaboration with patients' own expertise (the MI spirit)
   patient wisdom + support = patient-centered responsiveness

2. Proficiency in patient-centered counseling, including accurate empathy
   OARS
   Open-ended questions
   Affirmations (support self-efficacy; avoid argumentation)
   Reflective listening - verbal and nonverbal (develop discrepancy in patient)
   Summaries

   GROUP EXERCISE:
   In small groups, practice using the first two stages to further your understanding of verbal
    and nonverbal communication. In your group, one person will be the speaker, and two
   will be the reflectors (1 verbal/1 nonverbal). Select one of the following statements to
   discuss:
   a. Discuss your current struggles with motivational interviewing.
   b. If you could travel anywhere around the world, where would you go?
   c. How do you handle patient noncompliance?

3. Recognition of key aspects of patient speech that guide the practice of MI (recognizing and
reinforcing change talk)
   - evoke patient's motivation for change
   - minimize patient's resistance to discussing behavior change

4. Eliciting and strengthening patient change talk (building change talk)
   - use reflective, affirming, or elaborative statements based on patient speech
      In what ways would it be good for you to . . . .?
      If you did decide to . . . ., how would you do it?
      What would be the good things about . . . .?
      Why would you want to . . . .?
      What are the good things about . . .   And what are the not so good things?

GROUP EXERCISE:

<u>Case Study</u>

Lena is a community health center patient who presents with several health issues as a result of her smoking. At her last three visits to the center she met with her physician who repeatedly informed her that she needs to stop smoking in order to improve her health. Lena resists using any type of medicated support because she is afraid of the side effects, and continues to promise to "do better". She tries to stop on her own, but is finding difficulty overcoming her triggers. Her physician is frustrated at Lena's unwillingness to change.

What will you say to Lena? What is your plan for working with Lena?

5. Rolling with resistance (Ambivalence)

Patient: Well, I overeat it sometimes, but I don't have a problem with food.

Simple reflection: You don't think of yourself as a having a problem with food.

Amplified reflection: Your overeating has never really caused any problems or unpleasant effects in your life.

Double-sided reflection: You think you eat too much at times, and also you don't think of yourself as having a problem with food.

Miller and Rollnick (2002) recommend the following to address ambivalence:

• Make a statement indicating that you are reflecting the patient's perceptions of the issue, including any reasons or need for change noted by the patient.
• Summarize the patient's ambivalence, including the benefits of the current state of their situation.
• Provide objective evidence relevant to the importance of change.
• Restate patient's desire, ability, and commitment to change.
• Offer your assessment of the client's situation, especially when it matches the client's concern.

6. Negotiating change plans - timing is everything!
    SMART Goals
    Specific
    Measurable
    Achievable
    Realistic
    Timely

7. Consolidating patient commitment - based on patient's language of commitment
    "I will…", "I do…"
    On a scale from 0 to 10, how confident are you that you could . . . . .
    On a scale from 0 to 10, how important is it for you to . . . . .
    If you don't make any change, what do you think will happen?

    GROUP EXERCISE:
    Case Study Role Play:
    George is a Spanish-speaking patient with diabetes who visits the health center weekly

to check his blood sugar checked and review his dietary habits by a diabetes educator. A translator is brought in to sit with George and the diabetes educator to ensure that he understands the conversation. Each week the diabetes educator tells him each time that he could save himself some time if tests his blood sugar at home. He says,"¿No, no lo se, es muy dificil, verdad?" The educator gently insists that it is easy to do, and George seems to be receptive.

How do you use motivational interviewing techniques to offer advice to George?

What do you say to George when you are asking for:

Commitment to change

Setting specific goals

Development of a plan

Commitment to the plan

Internal readiness

A follow-up discussion, after the patient did not commit.

8. Switching flexibly between MI and other intervention styles (Intervention methods that support MI)

> Transtheoretical Stages of Change
> Precontemplation
> Contemplation
> Preparation
> Action
> Maintenance
> Relapse

GROUP EXERCISE:

Case Study

Donna is currently rehabilitating from knee replacement surgery, and shortly after discharge from the hospital she was readmitted for blood clots in her lungs. She was placed on Coumadin and informed that she needs to visit the health center weekly to monitor her health. Donna is concerned about her health, but despises the regiment of seeing a physician weekly. It takes her three weeks to start her first visit at the center. When told by the physician to return next week, Donna says, "I'll do my best, but I can't promise you." The physician responds, "Well, it's for your own good, but hey, that's up to you." Donna rolls her eyes and turns away.

How do you use motivational interviewing techniques to explore Donna's ambivalence?

Case Study

Martin is a nutritionist who runs a weekly class on healthy food choices and preparation for community health center patients. Many of the patients are reluctant to changing the recipes of their traditional meals, and Martin often struggles to get patients to attend. Those who do attend hesitate to try new foods. Martin sees that he needs to restructure his class to get a better turnout.

How do you use motivational interviewing techniques to assess patients' readiness for change?

Motivational Interviewing Strategies

There are specific strategies that are likely to elicit and support change talk in Motivational Interviewing:

1. **Ask Evocative Questions:** Ask an open question, the answer to which is likely to be change talk.
2. **Explore Decisional Balance:** Ask for the pros and cons of both changing and staying the same.
3. **Good Things/Not--So--Good Things:** Ask about the positives and negatives of the target behavior.
4. **Ask for Elaboration/Examples:** When a change talk theme emerges, ask for more details. "In what ways?" "Tell me more?" "What does that look like?" "When was the last time that happened?"
5. **Look Back:** Ask about a time before the target behavior emerged. How were things better, different?
6. **Look Forward:** Ask what may happen if things continue as they are (status quo). Try the miracle question: If you were 100% successful in making the changes you want, what would be different? How would you like your life to be five years from now?
7. **Query Extremes:** What are the worst things that might happen if you don't make this change? What are the best things that might happen if you do make this change?
8. **Use Change Rulers:** Ask: "On a scale from 1 to 10, how important is it to you to change [the specific target behavior] where 1 is not at all important, and a 10 is extremely important? *Follow up:* "And why are you at ___and not _____ [a lower number than stated]?" "What might happen that could move you from ___ to [a higher number]?" Alternatively, you could also ask "How confident are you that you could make the change if you decided to do it?"
9. **Explore Goals and Values:** Ask what the person's guiding values are. What do they want in life? Using a values card sort activity can be helpful here. Ask how the continuation of target behavior fits in with the person's goals or values. Does it help realize an important goal or value, interfere with it, or is it irrelevant?
10. **Come Alongside:** Explicitly side with the negative (status quo) side of ambivalence. "Perhaps _(ex. losing weight; stopping smoking)_____is so important to you that you won't give it up, no matter what the cost."

Adapted from:
http://www.motivationalinterview.org/Documents/1%20A%20MI%20Definition%20Principles%20&%20Approach%20V4%20012911.pdf

Motivational Interviewing Statements

Be sure to ask open-ended questions, listen attentively, and summarize what you heard.

Assess Readiness

Conventional Method	Motivational Interviewing Method
"I know you don't want to discuss _____, but I'm going to talk about with you."	"Would it be okay if we spent a few minutes discussing _____?"
"You need to address this health issue now."	"On a scale of 1 - 10, how important (or confident, or ready) are you to _____?"
"I'm sure this is difficult to deal with, but you need to consider how worse your health can get."	"Since now may not be the right time for you, what would need to happen for it to be the right time?"
"These are the steps you need to take to improve your health."	"What would you need to move from a 5 to a 7?"
"You really should follow what the doctor said."	"What would you like your next steps to be?"
When are you going to be ready to address this problem?	"I'm confident that if and when you make a decision and commitment to _____, you will do it."

Explore Ambivalence

Conventional Method	Motivational Interviewing Method
"If you don't change, your health will deteriorate."	"What are some of the advantages for keeping things just the way they are?"
"If you change, your health will improve."	"What would be some of the reasons for making a change?"
"Okay, what you need to do now is..."	"Let me see if I understand what you've said..."
"Okay, I got it all."	"Did I get all that you said?"

Offer Advice

Conventional Method	Motivational Interviewing Method
"My idea for how to handle your situation is _____"	"If you don't mind, I'd like to suggest an idea to think about. Would you like to hear it?"
"Let me tell you what you need to do...."	"May I share my experience? Based on my experience, I would encourage you to consider _____."
"As your provider, I'm telling you that you must do this."	"I completely understand that it's ultimately your choice."
"I think my suggestion would be the best decision for you."	"What do you think about that idea?"

Appendix

Case Studies with Model Responses

1. Lena is a community health center patient who presents with several health issues as a result of her smoking. At her last three visits to the center she met with her physician who repeatedly informed her that she needs to stop smoking in order to improve her health. Lena resists using any type of medicated support because she is afraid of the side effects, and continues to promise to "do better". She tries to stop on her own, but is finding difficulty overcoming her triggers. Her physician is frustrated at Lena's unwillingness to change.

What will you say to Lena? What is your plan for working with Lena?

Model Response: "If you don't mind, Lena, may I suggest a few ideas to consider that may help?"
[If she says no, then]:
"It seems that now may not be the right time for you to think about other options. What would need to happen for it to be the right time?"
[If she says yes, then]:
"Based on my experience, I would encourage you to consider _____. What do you think about that idea?"
[Lena's response should then guide her next steps toward smoking session.]

2. The waiting room is packed with patients, and Melissa has been waiting anxiously to see a nurse to discuss her next steps after receiving a diagnosis from the physician. Melissa speaks a little English, but Spanish is her primary language. The nurse finally sits with her to explain the types of treatments she can receive, and the series of appointments that must be set up over the next several weeks. Melissa sighs in frustration and says, "I can't deal with this right now. I really just can't handle it."

What will you say to Melissa? What is your plan for working with Melissa?

Model Response: "I'm hearing you say that you're not feeling able to handle it all, and possibly overwhelmed. It what ways?" or
"Please tell me more about what you are feeling."

3. Cynthia is a single mother with two children under 3. She had developed a comfort level with Maria, the receptionist at the community health center whom she often sees because of her children's frequent colds and ear infections. Today Cynthia is upset because Maria is not in and she has to speak with Tanya who is a new receptionist at the center.

What will you say to Cynthia? What is your plan for working with Cynthia?

Model Response: "How can I best assist you today?" or
"It what ways can I help you to have a productive visit today?"

4. Jenna has come to the center to see a physician because she notices a small lump in her breast. She is sent to get a mammogram right away. The technician assigned to her notices that Jenna is anxious and shaking as she prepares her for the screening. Jenna finally blurts out, "Please be gentle, and please tell me if you find anything!"

What will you say to Jenna? What is your plan for working with Jenna?

Model Response: "I applaud you for coming in for your mammogram. I will be as gentle as I can, just breathe as I talk you through the exam. I will answer as many questions as I can along the way, but the physician will provide you with the results of your mammogram. Before we get started please tell me a little more about what you're feeling now."

5. Robert is concerned about his HIV status and visits the center to get tested. He sits with the phlebotomist who is prepared to talk with Robert to ease his fears. Right before the phlebotomist is about to place the tourniquet on Robert's arm, he get's up and heads for the door saying, "I'm not ready to know my status. If I'm positive, what would I do?"

What will you say to Robert? What is your plan for working with Robert?

Model Response: "What are the worst things that might happen if you don't find out? What are the best things that might happen if you do find out?" or
"I applaud you for taking this step toward finding out about your status. If you are positive, I am confident that our center can provide you with enough resources to help you live a long healthy life." or
"I hear that you are hesitant about knowing your status. Tell me more about what you are feeling."

6. Steve is a community health center patient who comes frequently to get his high blood pressure checked by a CNA. The CNA notices that the often jovial and smiling Steve is somewhat melancholy. When the CNA takes his blood pressure, it reads higher than usual. When asked how he is feeling, Steve says, "What do you care? Just tell me my numbers."

What will you say to Steve? What is your plan for working with Steve?

Model Response: "I always care. It sounds like something is upsetting you. Do you want to talk

about what's upsetting you, Steve?" or
"I am here to listen, if you would like to talk, Steve"

7. George is a Spanish-speaking patient with diabetes who visits the health center weekly to check his blood sugar checked and review his dietary habits by a diabetes educator. A translator is brought in to sit with George and the diabetes educator to ensure that he understands the conversation. Each week the diabetes educator tells him each time that he could save himself some time if tests his blood sugar at home. He says,"¿No, no lo se, es muy dificil, verdad?" The educator gently insists that it is easy to do, and George seems to be receptive.

How do you use motivational interviewing techniques to offer advice to George?

Model Response: "If you don't mind, I'd like to suggest an idea to think about. Would you like to hear it?" or
"Based on my experience, I would encourage you to consider _____." or
"I completely understand that it's ultimately your choice." or
"What do you think about that idea?" [Then follow with]
"What are the best things that might happen if you do make this change?

8. Donna is currently rehabilitating from knee replacement surgery, and shortly after discharge from the hospital she was readmitted for blood clots in her lungs. She was placed on Coumadin and informed that she needs to visit the health center weekly to monitor her health. Donna is concerned about her health, but despises the regiment of seeing a physician weekly. It takes her three weeks to start her first visit at the center. When told by the physician to return next week, Donna says, "I'll do my best, but I can't promise you." The physician responds, "Well, it's for your own good, but hey, that's up to you." Donna rolls her eyes and turns away.

How do you use motivational interviewing techniques to explore Donna's ambivalence?

Model Response: "What are some of the advantages for keeping things just the way they are?" or
"What would be some of the reasons for making your weekly visits?" or
"Let's talk about your goals. What would you like to achieve and what would motivate you to get there? What would get in the way of you achieving your goals?"

9. Martin is a nutritionist who runs a weekly class on healthy food choices and preparation for community health center patients. Many of the patients are reluctant to changing the recipes of their traditional meals, and Martin often struggles to get patients to attend. Those who do attend hesitate to try new foods. Martin sees that he needs to restructure his class to get a better turnout.

How do you use motivational interviewing techniques to assess patients' readiness for change?

Model Response: "Would it be okay if we spent a few minutes discussing the types of foods you like to eat?" or
"What would you need to have happen for you to try new foods?" or
"How would you describe the foods you enjoy eating? How can we work together make small changes to your recipes to help you to enjoy your meals?" or
"How confident are you that you could make healthier food choices if you decided to do it?"

9 Tips for Motivational Interviewing Success

Express empathy (understanding and respect) to patient's concerns and needs.

Reflective listening is essential for validation of the patient's perspective.

The patient, not the professional, should present reasons for change, as well as benefits and concerns.

Avoid arguing for change.

New perspectives are suggested, not imposed.

Resistance from a patient is a signal to respond differently.

A patient's belief in the possibility of change is an important motivator.

The patient is responsible for choosing and carrying out change.

The professional's belief in the patient's ability to change becomes a self-fulfilling prophesy.

Addressing MI Resistance from Staff

- Explore reasons for resistance (eg. time, perceived value)

- Engage in dialogue about the pros and cons of Using MI

- Align benefits of MI with helping to improve work with patients

- Define management expectations and role model MI strategies

- Explore staff buy-in through the use of MI strategies (open-ended questions, affirmations, reflections, and ambivalence)

- Maintain an open dialogue and roll with resistance - refrain from power struggles

- Determine how to integrate MI with current methods of intervention

- Engage staff in MI trainings (and refresher trainings) that allow for pre/post discussion

Bibliography

Aharonovich, E., Greenstein, E., O'Leary, A., Johnston, B., Seol, S. G., & Hasin, D. S. (2012). HealthCall: Technology-based extension of motivational interviewing to reduce non-injection drug use in HIV primary care patients–a pilot study. *AIDS care*, *24*(12), 1461-1469.

Baidal, J. A. W., Price, S. N., Gonzalez-Suarez, E., Gillman, M. W., Mitchell, K., Rifas-Shiman, S. L., ... & Taveras, E. M. (2013). Parental Perceptions of a Motivational Interviewing–Based Pediatric Obesity Prevention Intervention.*Clinical pediatrics*, *52*(6), 540-548.

Carr, E. S., & Smith, Y. (2013). The Poetics of Therapeutic Practice: Motivational Interviewing and the Powers of Pause. *Culture, Medicine, and Psychiatry*, 1-32.

Haeseler, F., Fortin VI, A. H., Pfeiffer, C., Walters, C., & Martino, S. (2011). Assessment of a motivational interviewing curriculum for year 3 medical students using a standardized patient case. *Patient education and counseling,84*(1), 27-30.

Hardcastle, S., Blake, N., & Hagger, M. S. (2012). The effectiveness of a motivational interviewing primary-care based intervention on physical activity and predictors of change in a disadvantaged community. *Journal of behavioral medicine*, *35*(3), 318-333.

Hardcastle, S. J., Taylor, A. H., Bailey, M. P., Harley, R. A., & Hagger, M. S. (2013). Effectiveness of a motivational interviewing intervention on weight loss, physical activity and cardiovascular disease risk factors: a randomised controlled trial with a 12-month post-intervention follow-up. *International Journal of Behavioral Nutrition and Physical Activity*, *10*(1), 40.

Lozano, P., McPhillips, H. A., Hartzler, B., Robertson, A. S., Runkle, C., Scholz, K. A., ... & Kieckhefer, G. M. (2010). Randomized trial of teaching brief motivational interviewing to pediatric trainees to promote healthy behaviors in families. *Archives of pediatrics & adolescent medicine*, *164*(6), 561-566.

Mansyur, C. L., Pavlik, V. N., Hyman, D. J., Taylor, W. C., & Goodrick, G. K. (2013). Self-efficacy and barriers to multiple behavior change in low-income African Americans with hypertension. *Journal of behavioral medicine*, *36*(1), 75-85.

Mertens, V. C., Goossens, M. E., Verbunt, J. A., Köke, A. J., & Smeets, R. J. (2013). Effects of nurse-led motivational interviewing of patients with chronic musculoskeletal pain in preparation of rehabilitation treatment (PREPARE) on societal participation, attendance level, and cost-effectiveness: study protocol for a randomized controlled trial. *Trials*, *14*(1), 90.

Miller, W.R. & Moyers, T.B. (2007). Eight stages in learning Motivational Interviewing. *Journal of Teaching in the Addictions,* (5), 3-17.

Miller, W. R., & Rollnick, S. (2002). *Motivational interviewing: Preparing people for change* (2nd ed.). New York: Guilford Press.

Rollnick, S., & Miller, W. R. (1995). What is motivational interviewing?.*Behavioural and cognitive Psychotherapy, 23*(04), 325-334.

Miller, W. R., & Rose, G. S. (2009). Toward a theory of motivational interviewing. *American Psychologist, 64*(6), 527.

Naar-King, S., & Suarez, M. (2011). *Motivational interviewing with adolescents and young adults.* Guilford Press.

Price, S. N., McDonald, J., Oken, E., Haines, J., Gillman, M. W., & Taveras, E. M. (2012). Content analysis of motivational counseling calls targeting obesity-related behaviors among postpartum women. *Maternal and child health journal, 16*(2), 439-447.

Resnicow, K., & McMaster, F. (2012). Motivational interviewing: Moving from why to how with autonomy support. *International Journal of Behavioral Nutrition and Physical Activity, 9*(1), 19.

Russell, C. L., Cronk, N. J., Herron, M., Knowles, N., Matteson, M. L., Peace, L., & Ponferrada, L. (2011). Motivational Interviewing in Dialysis Adherence Study (MIDAS). *Nephrology Nursing Journal, 38*(3).

Söderlund, L. L., Madson, M. B., Rubak, S., & Nilsen, P. (2011). A systematic review of motivational interviewing training for general health care practitioners.*Patient education and counseling, 84*(1), 16-26.

Stawnychy, M., Creber, R. M., & Riegel, B. (2013). Using Brief Motivational Interviewing to Address the Complex Needs of a Challenging Patient With Heart Failure. *The Journal of cardiovascular nursing.*

Thompson, D. R., Chair, S. Y., Chan, S. W., Astin, F., Davidson, P. M., & Ski, C. F. (2011). Motivational interviewing: a useful approach to improving cardiovascular health?. *Journal of clinical nursing, 20*(9-10), 1236-1244.

VanBuskirk, K. A., & Wetherell, J. L. (2013). Motivational interviewing with primary care populations: a systematic review and meta-analysis. *Journal of behavioral medicine*, 1-13.

NOTES

NOTES

NOTES

www.ingramcontent.com/pod-product-compliance
Lightning Source LLC
Chambersburg PA
CBHW081757170526
45167CB00009B/4054